Healthy Living

i

Toxic World

Quick 'Lists & Tips'

Compiled from Hundreds of Sources

Mel Tavares

10.99

Healthy Living in a Toxic World

Quick Lists and Tips Reference Guide

ISBN-13: 978-1493612505

ISBN-10: 1493612506

This is the second revision and second printing of this book, expanded to include more information regarding GMO's.

Disclaimer: This book is in no way intended to be medical advice. Any reactions which may be caused by eating particular foods or using products are the liability of you, the reader, and not the author of the book. Any suggestions contained within this book which you follow, you are doing by choice and prescribing for yourself. The author has simply researched (General Resources listed at end of book) the subject matter, is applying the best practices to her own life, and is now sharing the information with you. This information is not a substitute for medical advice and does not in any way replace medical care.

DEDICATIONS

'Healthy Living in a Toxic World' is dedicated to my sister Lynn, who recently had a heart attack. It scared her and scared me enough to push me to finish this book and get it into the hands of all of us in need of clear and concise direction for healthy living. A special thanks to our Mom, who raised us to eat wholesome food, not junk.

It is also dedicated to all who have participated in the facebook support group (WE FIT) at any point over the past four years, and who continue to strive toward healthy living. If it were not for all of the sharing, encouragement, and yes-even chiding these past four years; I would have seen my health continue to decline. To each of you, I thank you! A shout-out to Brian, who clued me in, regarding foods that were causing inflammation.

Furthermore, this book is dedicated to Joanne; my former co-worker and friend, who had a major health scare and is now taking drastic steps to reverse the medical issues and reclaim her health.

Table of Contents

Contact Mel with questions or to request her to speak to your group.

Email: maryellensmith_rte@yahoo.com

Website: meltavares.com

Prologue

I am not skinny. There. That is out in the open. I want to be at a healthier weight and am working on that goal. I am also not a marathon runner. I don't have a degree in nutrition. I am just an ordinary person, struggling to figure out how to live healthy, in this ever increasingly toxic world.

I did not set out to write a book on the topic of healthy eating and living. I set out on this journey, in search of answers to why my own health was so poor and declining by the month. I grew up living rural. I have a degree in Horticulture/Agriculture, which I used professionally and personally. I raised and preserved my own food my entire life, until ten years ago.

It wasn't until I left the rural area of Maine and moved to urban Connecticut, that I started experiencing health issues and gaining unwanted pounds. Coincidence? As it turns out, no! There is a direct link between relocating from a rural community to a city. Now, my goal is to live urban with a rural mentality. AKA, a return to healthy living.

Once I began researching for answers to my own issues, I was stunned. Not only have I discovered some of the reasons for my own suffering, but also those of some friends and family members. One by one, I (and they) have begun implementing what I call 'best practices'. As I've done so, my symptoms are disappearing and my health is returning!

This is by no means an exhaustive book on the topic. Moreover, I feel that this is only the tip of the iceberg, just a glimpse of the toxic world we are living in and of the toxic 'food' and medicines we have all been consuming, and toxic products we have been using. The world we lived in 20 years ago is far different than the toxic world we live in now!

I could be selfish and just keep all of this researched information to myself, but I feel it would be wrong to do so. I recognize that not everyone is an accomplished researcher nor does everyone have the time to research and synthesize several hundred sites and books.

Therefore, **I am releasing my abridged findings to you**, in the most coherent and concise manner possible, in an easy to read and understandable format. I may release a more exhaustive book at a later date, but at this point, I want to give you the information so that you may begin to make informed choices, now.

This book contains truth and insight regarding our toxic world and how to stay healthy while living in it. The truths within this book are applicable to people in every country around the world. It crosses all ethnic and socio-economic barriers and gives bottom line information to the reader. As I said, I have taken hundreds of hours to synthesize several hundred books and sites I have read. *While the book may seem short and simplistic, the research behind it is anything but simplistic.*

Balance is the keyword. I am giving you the information, but realize that it would be a quantum leap for many to go from where you are now to using 100% all natural, totally certified organic products and practicing green living. The more urban of an area you live in, the more challenging it is going to be to live healthy in this toxic world. I am not there yet, and I realize the impossibility of getting to that point in the immediate future. I am, however, sure that I can continue to make changes in that direction. So can you.

A final note about this book: I was recently asked how I would keep this information updated. The answer is "I cannot." The information is current for early 2014, the timeline of the completion of this book. In the world we live in, updated information is available before a page can hardly be written. Therefore, if you find that information herein is no longer accurate, I ask that you please remember our fluid and rapidly changing world and use the resource sites listed as your basis for obtaining updated lists and information.

Mel Tavares

Principles to Live By

- Accept the reality that we don't know what we don't know. I have inadvertently, unwittingly fed my kids all the wrong foods, allowed them to consume sugars, bad carbs, and chemical/preservative filled foods. Move forward; armed with information, determine to improve your health.

- Cook primarily from 'scratch', and avoid pre-packaged products.

- If it's a plant, eat it. If it was made in a plant, don't eat it.

- If your food doesn't spoil, it's not fresh and chances are part of it is not even food.

- 80% of the food in the supermarket didn't exist 20 years ago! Shop the perimeter of the store, and buy few things from inside aisles. Before there were stores filled with man-made products, we got our foods from farms, forests, or fields!

- Drink water the majority of the time, and plenty of it.

- Buy organic when possible, that way you can avoid ingesting the nasty chemicals and pesticides often found on or in non-organic foods. If not possible, watch the labels and do the best you can.

- Eat/drink whole products-rather than fat free, sugar free, or skim products.

- Eat primarily fruits, veggies, nuts, and grains.

- Follow the 'eat healthy 80/20% of the time' principle.

- Cancer & infections cannot live in an alkaline body (eat greens, use lemons, drink water with cider vinegar in it).

- Eating healthy is the true 'detox diet'. There's nothing fancy about it, just some dedication and trust in the amazing functions of the human body.

- Exercise is #1 biochemical way to decrease stress. Exercising for 20 minutes., 4x a week is an effective anti-depressant.

- Attend to the underlying emotional issues and trauma that is causing you to turn to food for comfort.

- Sleep enough. Lack of sleep can increase weight.

- Visualize daily, how it will feel to be healthy and how you will look.

- Love much, yourself and others. Ditch toxic relationships and those who don't love you, your health depends on it.

- Live fully. Laugh much. Laughter is clinically proven to improve an immune system and decrease pain.

The Great Debate-GMO's

What does 'GMO' mean? GMO stands for genetically modified organism. In essence, the seed or plant has been genetically engineered and modified, to be resistant to weed killers and insecticides. The issue isn't within the seed itself, for the most part, but lies in the fact that the food is now treated with chemicals, as it is growing. The ramifications on a person's health are astronomical. More on that further along in this section.

A 2012 Mellman Group poll showed 91% of Americans want food labeled. CBS polls showed 53%. Either way, it is clear that Americans want policies similar to what most developed countries around the globe have embraced. Australia, Japan, the European Union and other countries have imposed an outright ban on GMO seeds and products, while multitudes more have put severe restrictions in place. They refuse to accept American GMO ridden exported seeds and foods. Americans are now demanding the same restrictions, if not an all-out ban on the GMO seeds and products being bioengineered and grown in their own back yards.

As you will read further along, you will discover it is not just the food crop itself that poses the problem, but the ingredients that are added to the food (say apples) when packaged as a whole food or when making a new product using various ingredients (think apple pie filling, frozen dinners). Furthermore, ingredients such as oil are made using GMO products and processing.

This past year has been one of continual victory for groups determined to enlighten the world about the impact of GMO's and the company responsible for genetic engineering.

A grassroots effort against the Missouri based company, Monsanto, has spread like wild fire. One woman whose passion was fueled by the failure of the state of California to require labeling of GMO food products, took it upon herself to begin organizing marches.

In May of 2013, hundreds of cities across the United States as well as many more across the globe, marched in protest of the mega company, Monsanto, and the practices utilized in producing food. That first march resulted in more than 2 million people banding together to demand changes be made.

Another march was held in the fall of 2013 and yet another in May of 2014. Each time, the number of marchers and participating cities around the globe increases. I recently met the organizer of the Providence, Rhode Island marches and she testified to the increasing awareness and refusal of citizens to continue accepting the status quo. Changes are eminent.

Monsanto's CEO, executives, and insiders have started dumping stock at an alarming rate as news of the danger of GMO's continues to spread across the globe like wildfire. As stock continues to plummet, victory chants are being heard around the globe.

GMO's are banned in 27 countries and food products must be labeled in an additional 61 countries, and the numbers are on the rise. After

Monsanto experiments contaminated nearby wheat fields in Oregon, USA recently, both South Korea and Japan banned imports on wheat from the US.

There is something amiss and the public is beginning to respond to the underhanded and highly-illegal contributions Monsanto is making, to buy power across the world.

Since 1999, Monsanto has contributed more than 380 million to the Whole Food Prize, in an effort to monopolize the world seed market and has expended millions more on advertising blitzes to refute the anti-GMO campaigns. El Salvador is the latest target of less than scrupulous tactics.

El Salvador banned the use of Monsanto seed in 2013. A year later, in June of 2014, the president of El Salvador became the recipient of the pressure exerted by Monsanto, to conform and buy the seed. Was it Monsanto, blatantly threatening the country of El Salvador? Oh, no! They are much too clever for that.

Michael Taylor, an appointee to the U.S. Food and Drug Administration is behind the attempt to get El Salvador to agree to purchase $277 million in seeds tainted with dozens of chemicals that are directly linked to pandemic increases of disease around the globe. Who is Michael Taylor? He is a former Vice President of-you guessed it-Monsanto! It is not likely a coincidence.

A study done by the European Union confirms the doom and gloom results of in-taking GMO's and has resulted in the Union enforcing even stricter food safety guidelines. Nevertheless, the US exerted pressure on Europe, in June of 2014, to ease the ban of bioengineered products. The European Union held its ground and did not succomb to the pressure.

What is all the fuss? Do GMO foods REALLY cause disease?
According to the Serailini GM Corn Rat study, 50% of males and 70% of females suffered premature deaths. Rats that ate GMO corn suffered an extremely high rate of tumors and organ damage. The list of consequences to a person's health is equally as long and becoming more evident with each passing month.

Here are just a few known side effects:

- Increased food allergies

- Body toxicity

- Increased reproductive issues and birth defects

- Increased issues with digestive system

- Obesity/'Wheat Belly' syndrome

- Heart Disease

- Kidney Disease

- Cancer

The war on GMO's is slowly being won. There are now hundreds of groups joining forces against the parent company, Monsanto and all of its subsidiaries. Large corporations, such as Whole Foods are responding with policies and promises to require accurate labeling of food products by 2018. That is four years from now. As groups continue to push for a faster policy change, alarms are being sounded at the grassroots level, informing consumers of action steps to take immediately, to avoid subjection to the harmful GMO's.

The US states of Maine and Connecticut were the first to pass conditional GMO labeling bills, paving the way for national policy changes. Chipotle Mexican Grill voluntarily disclosed the genetically modified ingredients on its menu, and other companies quickly followed suit. Consumer outrage over the information being publicized concerning health and environmental risks of GMO's, is at an all-time high.

I would be remiss to stop here and leave you feeling as I felt, when I began to research and read all of the information. I was overwhelmed. Discouraged. Defeated. Wondered what, on earth I could eat, that would be safe. I have taken my year of research and condensed it down to a few basic tips for avoiding GMO's in your food. *In order to succeed, you will need to become a vigilant label reader and a well-informed consumer.*

TIP #1: Look for "non-GMO" Labels

We are approaching a time when the mandate will exist for companies to label "Contains GMO's". Until then, you will have to read carefully. Companies may voluntarily label products as "non-GMO." Some labels state "non-GMO" while others spell out "Made without Genetically Modified Ingredients." Some products limit their claim to only one particular "At-Risk" ingredient such as soy lecithin, listing it as "non-GMO."

- Anything derived from genetically modified corn or soy, found in dozens of items, from the obvious corn and chips, soy protein or soy sauce, to the lesser known ingredients like dextrose or lecithin.

- Oils also contain GMO's, so avoid canola and cottonseed oil. If you're eating non-organic meat, eggs or dairy products, you are also eating the GMO grains they were fed. All sodas and HFCS sweetened soft drinks contain GMOs and the diet ones have questionable ingredients as well.

TIP #2: Avoid Sugar Products

Avoid all products with ingredients not listed as 100% cane sugar. GM sugar beets recently entered the food supply. Look for organic and non-GMO sweeteners, candy and chocolate products made with 100% cane sugar, evaporated cane juice, or organic sugar, to avoid GM beet sugar.

TIP #3:Know Your Numbers on UPC Codes

- <u>Organically Grown</u>: 5 digits, starting w/ no. 9

- <u>Conventionally Grown</u>: 4 digits, starting w/ no. 3 or 4

- <u>Genetically Modified</u>: 5 digits, starting w/ no. 8

TIP #4: Avoid products made with any crops that are known to primarily be GMO. The following is a list of ingredients to avoid.

Corn

Corn flour, meal, oil, starch, modified food starch, gluten, and syrup. Sweeteners such as fructose, dextrose, and glucose.

Soy

Soy flour, lecithin, protein, isolate, and isoflavone, vegetable oil and vegetable protein.

Canola

Canola oil

Cotton

Cottonseed oil

TIP #5: Buy Organic When Possible

"Certified Organic" products are not allowed to contain *any* GMOs. Therefore, when you purchase products labeled "100% organic" or "organic" all ingredients in these products are mandated to have been produced from GMO free crops.

Be aware: Products labeled as "made with organic ingredients" only require 70% of the ingredients to be organic, but 100% must be non-GMO. There are stories in the main stream news on a regular basis.

I know you may be thinking "I can't afford to eat organic." Later in the book, I will give you lists of which foods to buy organic, which foods are reasonably safe non-organic, and how to eat well on a budget.

A Word about the FDA and Food Recalls

If you are an American, or you live elsewhere but purchase food exported from America, you should be aware of potential dangers lurking in products. Beyond the concern over the millions of harmful foods and products the FDA has approved for human consumption and usage; is the concern of the agency needing to recall some of their approved products.

According to their website, "The FDA regulates products originating from more than 150 countries, 130,000 importers, and 300,000 foreign facilities. Fifty percent of fresh fruits, 20 percent of vegetables, and 80 percent of seafood consumed in America comes from abroad."

The reality is that the FDA cannot test each shipment that comes in, and often does not test unless there are complaints or reason for suspicion. In a 60 day period during the summer of 2013, the FDA recalled over 40 foods, the majority of which was not reported to consumers through major media outlets. Most know of the Chobani (Greek Yogurt) recall, but how many know of the recall of the others: recalled for containing undeclared peanuts, wheat, soy, milk, and other additives? Just this week, there was a massive recall in the northeast, of packaged salad mixes.

My conclusion remains the same. We cannot prevent 100% of diseases, in-taking tainted foods, or using harmful chemical based products. We can, however, drastically reduce consumption if we are properly educated. The internet provides immediate access to websites like the FDA. Learn to visit it, often.

Buying Pre-Packaged Foods

I encourage you to begin to purchase primary ingredients and prepare your own food. I do recognize, however, that time and talent does not always allow one to do so. You will find the following pages helpful in times when you are going to open a box, bag, or can.

A simple search on the internet will allow you to pull up a comprehensive list of companies who are certified non-GMO, those that offer some GMO products, and those known to be GMO based. Below are lists that I have compiled for my own usage, when buying packaged products. Please note that several companies offer both organic, non-GMO products as well as GMO laden products. **Watch your labels!**

GMO Free Brands

Author Note- *This list is simply a starting point, particularly for those still transitioning from buying pre-packaged to using whole foods.* I do not mean to infer these packaged products are better than whole foods or say that those below have been processed without some chemicals. You must still read the label to determine if the GMO free product is also organic. Remember that companies are ever changing, so what is true now-may not be true in 6 mos.

- Bob's Red Mill Organic
- Brown Cow Farm
- Cascadian Farms
- Earth's Best
- Eden
- Eggland's Best Organic
- Gerber
- Healthy Valley Organic
- Horizon Organic
- Jelly Belly

- Land O'Lakes Organic

- Lindt

- Luna

- Morningland Dairy

- Nature's Path

- Nest Fresh Organic

- Newman's Own (except salad dressings)

- Newman's Own Organics

- Odwalla

- Organic Baby

- Organic Valley

- Plum Organics

- Simply Nature

- Smuckers Simply 100% Fruit

- Sunridge Farms

- Stonyfield Farm

- Tasty Brand

- Vigoa Cuisine

- Woodstock Farms

Beware of Brands containing GMO's

Frankly, it is easier just to list 'safe' brands of pre-fab, processed foods! However, I am listing some (not all) of the primary labels in the global market-so that you recognize that your pantry and refrigerator may be full of GMO products. The exception is that in some countries, the brands use non-GMO ingredients. (Which causes us to wonder why they don't just offer the non-GMO product on a global scale. I digress.)

Be wary of most popular brands, as they may contain GMO's that are often found in products made with corn, soy, and other products.

- Aunt Jermima
- Beech-Nut
- Betty Crocker
- Bird's Eye
- Campbell's
- Capri Sun
- Chef Boyardee

- Coca-Cola

- Country Time

- Crystal Light

- Del Monte

- Dinty Moore

- Dole

- Duncan Hines

- Enfamil

- Gatorade

- General Mills

- Good Start

- Green Giant

- Hawaiian Punch

- Healthy Choice

- Heinz

- Hellmans

- Hersey's

- Hormel

- Hungry Jack

- Kellog's

- Kids Cuisine

- Kraft

- Lean Cuisine

- Libby's

- Lipton

- Marie Callenders

- Minute Maid

- Naked

- Near East

- Nestle

- Ocean Spray

- Pam

- Pepperidge Farms

- Peter Pan

- Pillsbury

- Post

- Power Bars

- Progresso Soups

- Quaker

- Similac

- Skippy

- Smuckers

- Sobe

- Sorrento

- Stouffer's

- Sunny Delight

- Swanson

- Tang

- Tropicana

- Wesson

- Wish Bone

Often, it is the **FOOD INGREDIENTS** which create GMO's on the aforementioned list of GMO brands. The ingredients are often created from GMO based products. There are exceptions, which can be found in products labels 100% organic. Again, you will have to read carefully, and research beyond what I am sharing here.

- Aspartame (also called NutraSweet®, Equal, Spoonful®, Canderel®, BeneVia®, E951)
- Canola oil
- Caramel color
- Cellulose
- Citric acid
- Cobalamin (Vit. B12)
- Colorose
- Condensed milk
- Confectioner sugar
- Corn flour
- Corn masa
- Corn gluten

- Corn meal

- Corn oil

- Corn sugar

- Corn syrup

- Cornstarch

- Cyclodextrin

- Cystein

- Dextrin

- Dextrose

- Diacetyl

- Diglyceride

- Erythritol

- Equal

- Food starch

- Fructose (any form)

- Glucose

- Glutamate

- Glutamic acid

- Gluten

- Glycerides

- Glycerin

- Glycerol

- Glycerol monooleate

- Glycine

- Hemicellulose

- High fructose corn syrup (HFCS)

- Hydrogenated starch

- Hydrolyzed vegetable protein

- Inositol

- Inverse syrup

- Invert sugar

- Inversol

- Isoflavones

- Lactic acid

- Lecithin

- Leucine

- Lysine

- Malitol

- Malt

- Malt syrup

- Malt extract

- Maltodextrin

- Maltose

- Mannitol

- Methylcellulose

- Milk powder

- Milo starch

- Modified food starch

- Modified starch

- Mono and diglyceride

- Monosodium

- Glutamate (MSG)

- Nutrasweet

- Poleic acid

- Phenylalanine

- Pytic acid

- Protein isolate

- Shoyu

- Sorbitol

- Soy flour

- Soy isolates

- Soy lecithin

- Soy milk

- Soy oil

- Soy protein

- Soy protein isolate

- Soy sauce

- Starch

- Stearic acid

- Sugar (unless cane)

- Tamari

- Tempeh

- Teriyaki marinade

- Textured vegetable protein

- Threonine

- Tocopherols (Vit E)

- Tofu

- Tehalose

- Triglyceride

- Vegetable fat

- Vegetable oil

- Vitamin B12

- Vitamin E

- Whey

- Whey powder

- Xanthan gum

Of the above listed, these are commonly agreed upon, to be the

10 Worst Ingredients in Food

Artificial Food Coloring

Aspartame (aka Nutrasweet etc)

BHA and BHT

High Fructose Corn Syrup (HFC)

Monosodium Glutamate (MSG)

Potassium Bromate

Recombinant Bovine Growth Hormone (rBGH)

Refined Vegetable Oil

Sodium Nitrate

Sodium Nitrite

The Health Impact of Chemicals in Our Food

It should come as no surprise to you there is a staggering impact on consumers, resulting from consuming chemical laden foods. Diseases that were almost unheard of 50 years ago are being diagnosed daily. Although the chemical additives are still legal, they are not healthy. The time has come to stop ignoring the problem and to take personal responsibility.

Heart Disease-The #1 Killer

Heart disease is a global issue. In the United States, heart disease is the leading cause of death. Statistics from the American Heart Association show that 75 million Americans currently suffer from heart disease, 20 million have diabetes and 57 million have pre-diabetes. These disorders are affecting younger and younger people in greater numbers every year. The reason I mention diabetes under heart disease is that the two are closely linked, and most people who are diabetic also suffer from heart disease.

Many think that heart disease is primarily an American disease. This is not correct thinking. According to the World Heart Federation, there are 17.3 million heart disease related deaths per year, globally. Of those, America makes up just under 2 million heart disease related deaths. The Western Pacific countries actually rank #1 with 4.7 million deaths a year and Europe ranks number 2 with 4.5 million. South East Asia ranks third, with 3.6 million. Only the Eastern Mediterranean and Africa rank lower than America, coming in at 1.3 million and 1.2 million, respectively.

Contrary to popular belief, heart disease is not just caused from high cholesterol, but also (and much more often) from the inflammation of blood vessels. What causes the chronic inflammation? **Quite simply, the overload of simple, highly processed carbohydrates (sugar, flour and all the products made from them) and the excess consumption of omega-6 vegetable oils like soybean, corn, and sunflower that are found in many processed foods.** Not coincidentally, this is a list similar to those listed in other sections of this book (e.g. chemical tainted, GMO laden products). Furthermore, the list is the same 'off limits list' given to diabetics!

Cancer-The #2 Killer

Globally, over 13 million people die of cancer per year. These numbers do not reflect the millions more who are currently battling the disease. Eastern Asia ranks 1st in death rates, North America second, Western Europe 3rd. The Caribbean, Africa, Northern Europe rank at the bottom of the global cancer death rate.

The World Cancer Report (WCR) indicates that the cancer rates could increase by 50%, to 15 million by 2020. The report reveals that cancer is perceived to be a major public health problem in developing countries.

This is not all due to smoking, as many would like to believe. **The majority of cases are attributed to people living an unhealthy lifestyle.** This includes consuming processed, chemical filled foods, environmental toxins, toxins in health and beauty products, and in cleaning agents.

What was once considered a "Western Disease" is now of deep concern, as more developing countries gain access to the western lifestyle. According to the WCR, stomach, and colon cancer are amongst the most common malignancies. **The report says that consuming just 1 pound of fresh fruits and vegetables per day can reduce the risk of cancer by up to 25%.** Drastically reducing or eliminating processed foods decreases risks even further, and switching to organic health and home products nearly eradicates the individual risk.

200 diseases and conditions

Disease prevention seems pretty straight-forward. There is an endless stream of information available to each of us, speaking in depth to what I have merely touched on in the preceding pages.

We have no lack of information and most of us understand the bottom line. Eat as pure, clean, whole, and organic as you possibly can. Educate yourself on what essential vitamins and minerals you need to keep your body functioning properly, to prevent over 200 diseases and conditions. Move your body. Use organic health and beauty products. Avoid medications when at all possible. Prevention is the best route, and healthy food is the best medicine. Clean 'as green' as possible.

Here is just a partial list of diseases and conditions, directly linked to not adhering to the above stated lifestyle. Disclaimer: I am not saying that that lifestyle can prevent disease 100% of the time. Obviously, other factors exist. What I <u>am</u> saying is that <u>many</u> of the conditions or diseases can be prevented, improved, or eliminated with a healthy lifestyle.

- Acid Reflux Disease (GERD)

- Acne

- Allergies

- Antisocial Personality Disorder

- Attention Deficit Disorder (ADHD/ADD)

- Altitude Sickness

- Alzheimer's

- Arthritis

- Asthma

- Back Pain

- Baldness

- Bedwetting

- Bladder Cancer

- Bone Cancer

- Brain Cancer

- Breast Cancer

- Brain Tumors

- Bronchitis

- Burns

- Bursitis

- Cancer

- Canker Sores (Cold Sores)

- Carpal Tunnel Syndrome (CTS)

- Celiac Disease

- Cervical Cancer

- Cholesterol

- Chronic Obstructive Pulmonary Disease (COPD)

- Colon Cancer

- Congestive Heart Failure (CHF)

- Cradle Cap

- Crohn's Disease

- Dandruff

- Deep Vein Thrombosis (DVT)

- Dehydration

- Depression

- Diabetes

- Diaper Rash

- Diarrhea

- Diverticulitis

- Drug Abuse

- Dyslexia

- Ear Infections

- Ear Problems

- Eating Disorders

- Eczema

- Eye Problems

- Fibromyalgia

- Gallbladder Disease

- Gallstones

- Generalized Anxiety Disorder (GAD)

- Gout

- Gum Diseases

- Headache

- Heart Attacks

- Heart Disease

- Heartburn

- Heat Stroke

- Heel Pain

- Hives

- Hyperglycemia (High Blood Sugar)

- Hyperkalemia (High Potassium)

- Hypertension (High Blood Pressure)

- Hyperthyroidism

- Hypothyroidism

- Infectious Diseases

- Infectious Mononucleosis (Glandular Fever)

- Influenza

- Infertility

- Insulin Dependent Diabetes Mellitus (IDDM)

- Iron Deficiency Anemia

- Irritable Bowel Syndrome (IBS)

- Itching

- Joint Pain

- Juvenile Diabetes

- Juvenile Rheumatoid Arthritis (JRA)

- Kidney Diseases

- Kidney Stones

- Leukemia

- Liver Cancer

- Lung Cancer

- Mesothelioma

- Migraine

- Muscle Cramps

- Muscle Fatigue

- Muscle Pain

- Neck Pain

- Obesity

- Osteoarthritis (OA)

- Osteomyelitis

- Osteoporosis

- Ovarian Cancer

- Ovarian Cyst

- Pain

- Panic Attack

- Phobias

- Pink Eye (Conjunctivitis)

- Pneumonia

- Post Nasal Drip

- Premenstrual Syndrome (PMS)

- Prostate Cancer

- Psoriasis

- Renal Failure

- Scabies

- Scars

- Sinus Infections

- Skin Cancer

- Skin Rash

- Sleep Apnea

- Sleep Disorders

- Stomach Cancer

- Strep Throat (Sore Throat)

- Sunburn

- Testicular Cancer

- Tooth Decay

- Tuberculosis (TB)

- Ulcers

- Urinary Tract Infection (UTI)

- Varicose Veins

- Vertigo

- Warts

- Yeast Infection (Candidiasis)

A Dozen 'Disease Causing Foods' You Should Work on Eliminating From Your Diet

- White Breads/Refined Flours

  Sidebar: Statistically, there is more gluten in a single slice of bread now than there was in 9 slices just a decade ago! Translated, that means that when you eat a sandwich, you are consuming as nearly as much gluten as was in an entire loaf of bread-10 years ago! No wonder people have issues with gluten! Any of us who sat down and ate a loaf of bread 'back in the day' would have been pretty sick then, also! Add several dozen chemicals to that loaf of bread and disaster (and disease) is eminent.

- Sugar filled Foods and Drinks

- Frozen Meals-Except Organics

- White Rice

- Microwave Popcorn

- Deli Meats, Hotdogs, Sausage, Bacon (Nitrates)

- GMO Foods

- Margarine

- Soy and Soy-based Products

- Diet 'anything'

- Pre-Packaged 'anything'

- Canned Items

Food as Medicine

Prevention of disease is far better than having to heal from it. Nonetheless, healing from the disease is far better than living with it- or dying from it. Food should be a healing agent to our bodies. If we eat the correct foods and are careful to increase or decrease particular ones, based on our current health status, there is a high probability that our bodies will repair themselves.

The cells in our bodies are constantly dividing, regenerating, and dying, but each cell's life cycle is different. The cells lining the stomach, because they're exposed to acid, replace themselves about every five days. Cells in the epidermis last about a week. Red blood cells live for approximately four months in the body. Some cells take much longer to regenerate. A bone completely remodels itself and replaces its cells every seven years or so.

Why do I tell you this? Because, it gives <u>hope</u>. Knowing that your body is reproducing cells on a continual basis should convince you that you can <u>feed your body good foods while eliminating chemical laden foods,</u> and *see major results in under six months!* Many diseases can be completely eradicated from the body by simply feeding it correctly and eliminating harmful toxins!

Elsewhere, I listed foods that are healthy, and included herbs and spices on the list. Below is a partial list of the specific benefits that various ones offer. To receive full benefit, try to incorporate as many of these as possible into your daily cooking routine.

Beneficial Herbs and Spices

- <u>Apple Cider Vinegar</u>- Eliminates bad breath, headaches, fatigue, varicose veins, arthritis, infections, soothes bug bites, regulates PH in body, aids in wt. loss by breaking down fats, helps prevent acne, gets rid of warts, prevents flu and stomach viruses, dissolves kidney stones.

- <u>Basil</u>-De-stresses, clears skin disorders.

- <u>Blueberries</u>-fight bladder infections, improves memory.

- <u>Cacao-raw chocolate</u>-use to bake with, add to drinks, or nibble on-not the 'other' chocolate.

- <u>Cayenne Pepper</u>-Metabolism, fights flu, relieves fatigue, relieves arthritis symptoms, fibromyalgia, nerve pain.

- <u>Chia seeds</u>-one of best foods. It binds toxins and causes them to move through the digestive tract, provides calcium, vitamins, is a protein food that aids in preventing cancer, anti-inflammatory, boosts immune, provides energy, relieves joint pain, stabilizes blood sugar and more.

- <u>Cinnamon</u>-Metabolism, Fights Flu, #1 blood sugar regulator and diabetes fighter, also fights the bacteria that causes yeast infections throughout body, anti-inflammatory, also cures stomach ulcers, prevents colon cancer, relieves constipation, improves memory, and acts as a blood thinner-heart health.

- <u>Cinnamon & Honey</u>: fights cold, flu, cancer, heart disease, bladder infections, upset stomach, relieves toothaches (rub on gums)…use externally to get rid of acne.

- <u>Cloves</u>- Fights flu and other diseases.

- <u>Coconut Oil</u>-very very long list of benefits (can extract it at home, jar the oil, use the 'meat')-Improves just about every body function there is!

- <u>Coffee</u>-boosts metabolism, thwarts migraines.

- <u>Cranberries</u>-prevent Urinary Tract Infections.

- <u>Dill</u>-Metabolism booster.

- <u>Flax seed</u>- Long list of benefits (do the research). Once vacuum seal on milled is broken, *shelf life is 3 mos. Buy small quantities* only. Soak the seeds in water (to release the nutrition); then slow roast in oven to create granola. Eat as breakfast cereal. Mix some in yogurt. Add it to smoothies or stir some into juice.

- <u>Garlic</u>-Kidneys, metabolism, kills cancers (virtually ALL types if used daily-only a couple types if used a two or three times a week), lowers cholesterol, natural antibiotic-fights infection, boosts immune system, maintains proper blood pressure, B6 vitamin, inflammation fighter, pain reliever.

- <u>Ginger</u>- Fights flu, migraines, inflammation, arthritis symptoms, cold symptoms, colon/ovarian cancer. 'Candies' are a great alternative to cough drops.

- <u>Horseradish-</u> has many benefits, including correcting sinus issues.

- <u>Lemon Zest (orange also)</u> (peels have 5x more vitamins than the juice)-prevents cancer, infections, increases bone health, regulates blood pressure, is an anti-depressant, prevents cysts and tumors.

- <u>Mint</u>-Metabolism, eliminates bad breath.

- <u>Olive Oil</u>-Skin complexion, brain functioning.

- <u>Onions</u>-Kidneys, fights flu.

- <u>Oregano</u>-Metabolism, antioxidants (1 t. = 3 CUPS of broccoli!).

- <u>Parsley</u>-Kidneys, metabolism, eliminates bad breath, heart health, fights cancer, balances blood pressure, ear infections and ringing in ears.

- <u>Raw Honey</u>-(if it is processed, it loses its vitamins, and ability to do the following): Fights flu, fights allergies, aids digestion, improves heart health, fights diabetes by stabilizing blood sugar, Natural Vit. B complex-lowers stress, antioxidant, immune booster, increases metabolism-therefore burns fat, fights fatigue. Use it for mouth sores.

- <u>Rosemary</u>-Anti-inflammatory, heart health, prevents breast cancer and skin cancer.

- <u>Tomatoes</u>-fights cancer by capturing free radicals, aid in fighting leg cramps.

- <u>Thyme</u>-Antioxidant, improves respiratory function.

- <u>Turmeric</u>- Fights flu, kills cancer, anti-inflammatory-India uses
  in nearly every meal! Jamaican beef patties have added turmeric
  to the flour.

- <u>Water</u>-keeps all systems working correctly, aids in quick repair
  of muscle injuries.

Water is Essential

You <u>NEED</u> Water!!! Your body composition:

Brain-is 74.5 % water

Muscles-76% water

Bones-22% water

Fat-20% water

Skin-70% water

Connective Tissue-60% water

Kidneys-83% water

Liver-86% water

Blood-83% water

- SPRING Water is better than the purified. Unfiltered city water is very bad for you, due to chlorine and other chemicals and bacteria.

- Reduces risk of stroke and heart attack by 41%, a glass before meals aids digestion, a glass of warm water and lemon in a.m. aids organs to begin functioning, gives energy because not dehydrated, reduces risk of bladder and colon cancer by nearly 50%, boosts metabolism, balances PH to alkaline.

- Add Lemons (or Limes) -Detoxes, boosts immune system, cleanses blood, flushes liver and kidneys, removes radiation from body, suppresses appetite, makes hair shine and stronger, strengthens bones, controls blood pressure, boosts metabolism.

Rule of thumb for calculating how much water to consume daily: weigh yourself, divide # in ½, and drink that # of ounces. If doing cardio-add 8 oz. for every 20 minutes you exercise. If drinking caffeine-add 8 oz., as well, for every 8 oz. of caffeine

consumed.

Need something more than water to drink?

- Peppermint tea (double strength) or Chamomile Great for headaches, especially during detox. Buy organic.

- Emergen-C is a holistic electrolyte replacement-drink it mixed in water, instead of Gatorade (3x a day will help with fatigue and muscle cramping).

- Rooibos Tea-Better than green tea! It is actually a root, not tea at all! More anti-oxidants and combats sugar cravings.

- Black and green tea-fight cancer by halting division of cancer cells. Chai tea is the best choice, because it has many of the above listed spices in it also, giving added health benefits.

- Dark Roasted Coffee-buy organic, non-processed when possible.

Top Artery Cleansing Foods

- Apples

- Asparagus

- Avocado

- Broccoli

- Brown Rice

- Cheese

- Cherries

- Cinnamon

- Coffee *2-4 cups a day

- Cranberries

- Garbanzo Beans

- Garlic *1-4 cloves a day

- Grapefruit

- Grapes

- Green Tea

- Nuts

- Oatmeal

- Olive Oil

- Orange Juice

- Pomegranate

- Spinach

- Strawberries

- Sweet Potatoes

- Tomatoes

- Watermelon

- Salmon

- Tumeric

Top Cancer Fighting Foods

- Acai Berries

- Avocados

- Beet Greens

- Berries (organic/wild)

- Broccoli

- Cabbage

- Cauliflower

- Chili Peppers

- Dandelion Greens

- Figs

- Flax Seed

- Garlic

- Ginger

- Ginseng

- Grapefruits

- Green Juice

- Herbal Green Tea

- Jalapenos

- Kale

- Lemons

- Mustard Greens

- Peaches

- Pomegranate

- Romaine Lettuce

- Rosemary

- Seaweed

- Swiss Chard

- Spinach

- Tomatoes

- Tumeric

Top Memory Building Foods

- Almonds

- Apples

- Blueberries

- Broccoli

- Brussel Sprouts

- Cabbage

- Cantaloupe

- Cauliflower

- Ginger

- Lettuce

- Pine Nuts

- Walnuts

- Watermelon

Health Issues Associated with Low Magnesium

- Cardiovascular –irregular heartbeats, heart attacks, high blood pressure, heart palpitations, angina.

- Digestive-constipation, difficulty swallowing.

- Genitourinary-kidney stones, urinary spasms.

- Gynecological/Reproductive: Menstrual cramps, pregnancy induced hypertension (high blood pressure), PMS, miscarriage.

- Metabolic-carbohydrate intolerance, insulin resistance, low calcium, low potassium, elevated phosphorous, vitamin D resistance.

- Musculoskeletal-muscle cramps, muscle soreness, muscle tension, muscle spasms/tremors, restless leg syndrome.

- <u>Neurological</u>-chronic fatigue, hearing loss, ringing in ear, vertigo, hyperactivity, restless children, insomnia, migraines, sinus headaches, nervous tension, numbness, tingling, persistent buzzing in ear.

- <u>Mental</u>-Anxiety, depression, irritability, panic attacks.

- <u>Other</u>-acute wheezing, allergy flare-ups, bronchitis, chemical sensitivities, chest tightness, chocolate cravings, craving carbs, craving salt, fibromyalgia, sensitivity to bright lights, sensitivity to loud noise.

Magnesium Rich Foods

- Almonds

- Basil

- Brazil Nuts

- Broccoli

- Cacao

- Chives

- Dill

- Flax Seeds

- Okra

- Pine Nuts

- Pumpkin Seeds

- Sesame Seeds

- Spearmint

- Spinach

- Sunflower Seeds

- Watermelon Seeds

Food as a Natural Pain Remedy (The Short List)

- Almonds for Headaches

- Blueberries for bladder infections

- Coffee for Migraines

- Cranberries for UTI infections

- Flax seed for breast pain and soreness

- Honey for mouth sores

- Horseradish for sinus

- Tomato juice for leg cramps

- Turmeric for chronic pain

- Water for injuries

Flushing Toxins Out of Your Body

Everyone has some level of toxins in their body. The question is, how much do YOU have in yours? Statistics show that the average person walking around has between 2 and 25 pounds of toxins in their body! That is downright disgusting, when we sit and think about it.

What do I mean by toxins? Toxins are trapped chemicals and byproducts that are a result of eating the wrong foods and drinking the wrong drinks; combined with not eating enough of the right ones.

The good news is that you can flush the toxins out of your body, beginning today, and will start feeling better within just a few short days. Earlier in the book, I mentioned over 200 diseases and conditions that are the cause of poor habits and intake of food. Many of them are caused, initially, by the toxins that are in our system. Take away the toxins, put your body back into right standing nutritionally, and the majority of health issues will disappear!

As I said in that section of the book, this is by no means a guarantee that your current condition will reverse, or a guaranteed prevention of the onset of future health issues. It is however, very likely that you will see a radical change for the better, and there are websites and books filled with testimonies from people who have seen a full cure/reversal in their medical conditions, simply by changing their lifestyle 180 degrees! If you do nothing, I will guarantee this-you are far more likely to see no improvement and are very likely to continue to experience an unexplained decline in your health.

Take the first step. Begin to flush the toxins out of your body. The following pages outline some simple steps you can take.

3 Simple Steps for Flushing Toxins

The concept of doing a detox is where most people cringe and get turned away, but it is a very simple and effective way to flush toxins out of your body.

1. Eliminate processed foods

2. Eat whole/raw fruits and veggies, and limited lean meats

3. Drink one or two cups of 'tea' a day.

Here is the 'tea' recipe that I use.

* 1 thick slice of lemon

*1 Tablespoon of honey

* 1 piece of fresh ginger, 2/3" long, peeled and bruised

* 1 cup boiling (purified) water

Place lemon and ginger in a cup, add boiling water and leave to infuse for two minutes. Remove lemon and ginger. Add honey and drink. *Note, I often use ground ginger in place of the ginger root, and sometimes use lemon juice instead of a lemon. Of course, the real deal is better, but a substitute is better than nothing!

More Tips For Detoxing

- Use <u>Chia Seeds</u> Daily. As they move through intestines, they will absorb and bind toxins including bile salts from liver.

- Eat <u>Parsley</u> often. It cleanses your blood supply, thereby cleaning the toxins from the blood.

- Cook with <u>Cilantro</u>. It binds heavy metals, especially mercury, which is a neurotoxin found in fish and dental work.

- <u>Broccoli sprouts</u> are super high in antioxidants that help detox enzymes in the digestive tract.

- <u>Vitamin C</u> is one of the best detox vitamins around, so it's no surprise lemons, oranges and limes made our list. The enzymes help to clear the digestive tract and cleanse the liver.

- <u>Garlic</u>-adding raw or cooked garlic to your food helps to filter out residual toxins.

- <u>Green Tea</u>-This well-known tea washes out toxins with its special antioxidants called catechism, which also increase liver function.

Tips for Improving Beauty, Naturally

- The cosmetic industry is a toxic dumping ground and WILL cause disease and health complications. Consider buying alternative products.

- Leisurely walks and bike rides are important. Strive for 20 minutes a day if leading a predominately sedentary lifestyle. Strenuous exercise actually counteracts weight loss attempts, as it signals the body to store/reserve fat for energy to use during exercise, so all the hard work of eating right-is actually counteracted. Exercise will rid the body of toxins, such as BPA residue.

- Take a hot bath in Epsom salts. It will serve as a major detox.

- Acne Fighting Tips: Avoid simple carbs, flour products; skip sugars, artificial sweeteners, and preservatives; and stay hydrated!

- Use a brush to do dry skin brushing. Removing dead skin cells which is important to keep them from clogging the system and will also help improve skin texture. Dry skin brushing can also boost the immune system and reduce the duration of infections or illness by removing toxins quicker as well as stimulating the lymph system to move waste matter out.

Striking a Balance

Phasing Out the Old, Phasing In the New

I can't say that I have successfully phased out every single processed food from my weekly intake, and I'd be lying if I said I never eat out. What I can say is that after a year of concerted effort, I am eating primarily whole foods, a majority of which are in keeping with the guidelines of this book. I confess that my biggest struggle is eliminating the bad carbs, specifically- white flour products. I can say that my eating habits do not remotely resemble those of a year ago, and I am conscious of every one of the attributes of food or drink that I consume.

Extremely overweight people were 70% less likely to develop diabetes when they lost just 5% of their weight, even if they didn't exercise. If you weigh 175 pounds, that's a little less than 9 pounds! I read this statistic and was spurred on to work to lose the 5% suggested to be necessary.

German researchers found that 1 gram of cinnamon a day helped adults with type 2 diabetes reduce their blood sugar by 10%. Why? Compounds in cinnamon may activate enzymes that stimulate insulin receptors. Other parts of this book have listed additional benefits of using cinnamon. I integrate cinnamon into my daily diet, and am confident that I am reaping multiple benefits.

Exercise, even if it's not for the purpose of losing weight. A Nurses' Health Study, for example, found that women who worked up a sweat more than once a week reduced their risk of developing diabetes by 30%! The reason? When you're stressed, your body is primed to take action. This gearing up causes your heart to beat faster, your breath to quicken, and your stomach to knot. But it also triggers your blood sugar levels to skyrocket. I can't say that I enjoy exercise. I can say that I make myself do it a couple times a week, at least.

Basic Health Guidelines

Here are some of the strategies that I have implemented and am happy to report are working!

- Eat a healthy diet, as outlined in this book and resource sites.

- Replace sweetened drinks (sugar or artificial sugars) with water.

- Avoid GMO products.

- Consume healthy fats.

- Eat plenty of raw foods.

- Exercise regularly.

- Get at least ½ hour of sunlight a day, without sunscreen.

- Limit toxin exposure in the environment.

- Get plenty of sleep.

- Manage your stress.

Friendly Reminder

Most of us have been consuming fake foods our entire lives. Changing our lifestyle to consume 100% high-nutrient foods is especially crucial if we want to reverse years of damage already done within our bodies. If you feel like this is an unattainable, impossible goal, drop the standard to a lower percentage (50-50 or 80-20). One thing is for certain. Even minor changes can often lead to major results. You have nothing to lose except poor health, by taking some steps in the right direction.

Food Shopping as a Health Conscious Consumer

There is a common belief that eating healthy is boring. Below is a list of 'real foods', many of which have endless varieties (e.g. apples), leaving the buyer with over 200 food choices. In simplest terms, real food is food you can imagine growing in nature; something our great-grandparents would recognize.

Once whole foods have been purchased, there are myriads of ways to prepare and/or combine foods. This leaves you, the consumer, with literally thousands of meal options!

Allow yourself to enjoy your favorite foods mindfully. When possible, eat the expensive, best quality version-organic is best (e.g. top quality ice cream, grass fed beef, free range chicken).

Shopping can be a hassle, which is why many of us tend to order out, go through a drive-through, or just grab a convenience product. The following lists can be helpful. Keeping non-perishable foods and spices on hand makes life less of a hassle, as many of them need to be bought at health food stores or larger grocery stores.

Tip: Online shopping direct from companies or through Amazon is a great way to save both time and money. In my region, I can shop online at peapod.com and have perishable and non-perishable grocery items delivered to my door for a $9.95 charge for orders under $100 and only $6.95 for orders over $100!

Tip: There are thousands of Aldi food stores, worldwide. Aldi now carries 'Simply Nature' and other labels, which offer GMO free and/or organic products. On average, these labels run .50 higher than a similar product of a different label but are MUCH cheaper than going to a specialty store.

Remember, the best way to ensure a healthy diet is to use the recommended food lists as <u>ingredients</u> in raw or cooked meal preparation, for juicing, or to eat as stand-alone foods.

Tip: Track your food intake for a week and then check to see how much variety you are getting into your diet! Make adjustments the following week. You will be surprised how quickly you can start eating healthier!

Dirty Dozen (Plus) *These are the ones you should definitely*

buy organic!

- Apples
- Celery
- Cherry Tomatoes
- Corn
- Cucumbers
- Grapes
- Hot Peppers
- Kale/Collard Greens
- Peaches
- Potatoes
- Spinach
- Strawberries
- Summer Squash

- Sweet Bell Peppers

A-Z List of Whole Foods and Spices (A compilation

of all lists aforementioned in this book. Please remember to

cross-reference this list with others (i.e. the Dirty Dozen, for

example).

Partaking of a wide variety of the foods on this list on a weekly basis

ensures that you are eating foods that are super foods, cancer

fighters, insulin controllers, digestion aids, heart healthy, magnesium

rich, anti-inflammatory, metabolism boosters, natural pain killers,

high fiber, natural detoxifiers, memory builders, and more!

- Acai Berries
- Almonds
- Apples
- Apple Cider Vinegar (Raw)
- Artichoke
- Asparagus
- Avocados
- Basil
- Bananas
- Barley

- Beans (all types)

- Beef

- Beet Greens

- Beets

- Blackberries

- Black Pepper

- Blueberries

- Brazil Nuts

- Broccoli

- Brussel Sprouts

- Buckwheat

- Butter

- Cabbage

- Cacao

- Cantaloupe

- Carrots

- Cashews

- Cauliflower

- Cayenne Pepper

- Celery

- Cheeses

- Cherries

- Chia Seeds

- Chicken

- Chick Peas

- Chili Peppers

- Chives

- Cilantro

- Cinnamon

- Cloves

- Coconut

- Coconut Oil

- Coffee

- Collard Greens

- Corn (Organic)

- Cranberries

- Cream

- Cucumbers

- Curry

- Dandelion Greens

- Dates

- Dill

- Eggplant

- Eggs

- Figs

- Fish

- Flax Seed (or Oil)

- Garbanzo Beans

- Garlic

- Ginger

- Ginseng

- Grapefruit

- Grapes

- Greek Yogurt

- Green Juices

- Green Tea

- Honey

- Horseradish

- Jalapenos

- Kale

- Kiwi

- Leeks

- Lemon

- Lentils

- Lime

- Lettuce (Esp. Romaine)

- Mango

- Maple Syrup

- Millet

- Milk

- Mint

- Molasses

- Mushrooms

- Mustard

- Mustard Greens

- Nuts

- Oats

- Okra

- Olive Oil

- Onions

- Oranges

- Oregano

- Paprika

- Papaya

- Parsley

- Passion Fruit

- Peaches

- Pears

- Peas (fresh or dried)

- Peanut Butter

- Peanuts

- Pears

- Pineapple

- Pine Nuts

- Plums

- Pomegranate

- Potatoes

- Prunes

- Pumpkin (and seeds)

- Quinoa

- Radishes

- Raisins

- Raspberries

- Rice (Brown or Basmati)

- Rice Noodles

- Rosemary

- Rye

- Salmon

- Sea Salt

- Seaweed

- Shellfish

- Spearmint

- Spinach

- Strawberries

- Sesame Seeds

- Spelt

- Squash (all types)

- Sunflower Seeds

- Sweet Potatoes

- Swiss Chard

- Tea (herbal, green, or black)

- Thyme

- Tomatoes

- Tumeric

- Turkey

- Vanilla (pure)

- Watermelon (and seeds)

- Walnuts

- Water

- Wild Game

- Whole Wheat

- Yams

Tips for Purchasing 'GMO Free' Snacks

You are hungry and forgot to pack snacks. Here is a partial listing of brands that offer GMO free options. Remember <u>not all non-GMO products are 100% organic.</u> Read your labels. Regardless of whether 100% organic or not, the goal is to make a <u>better choice</u> than grabbing a bag of orange cheese balls or a snack cake that has a shelf life of 50 years! (Such as is the case with my former favorite options).

- Angie's Artisan Treats
- Annie's
- Arrowhead Mills
- Attune
- Bakery on Main
- Barbaras
- Barefruit
- Beanitos
- Bites of Bliss

- Black Jewel

- Boulder Canyon Natural Foods

- Brad's Raw

- Ciao Bella

- Doctor in the Kitchen

- Earth's Best

- Eat Pastry

- Eden

- Garden of Eatin'

- Good Health

- Home Free

- Just Fruit

- Kettle

- Kettle Pop

- Koyo

- La Tolteca

- Live.Love.Snack

- Mary's Gone Crackers

- Mediterranean Organics

- Nature's Bakery

- Nature's Path

- New England Natural Bakers

- Peeled Snacks

- Popcornopolis

- Que Pasa

- Simply Nature

- Simply 7

- Snikkidy

- Sunridge Farms

- Taste of Nature

- Trees of Life

- Udi's

Top Ten Best Fast Food Options

You know and I know that we live in a fast paced world. Most of us have days that we are not going to cook. Say what we will about healthy living and eating, there is still the 80/20 rule that I mentioned earlier in the book. Below is the list of the best choices if you are using the 'drive through' for a quick meal.

- Arby's-Ham & Cheese

- Burger King- Double Hamburger

- Chinese-Steamed Vegetables and Spring Roll

- KFC- Grilled Chicken Breasts

- McDonalds-Chicken Caesar Salad

- Sonic-Grilled Chicken Wrap

- Starbucks- Steel Cut Oatmeal with Fruit

- <u>Subway</u>-Oven Roasted Chicken Salad *(At the time this book was preparing to go to press, Subway announced their intent to reformulate their bread recipes, following pressure exerted by more than 50,000 petitioners who demanded the chemical azodicarbonamide, be removed)*

- <u>Taco Bell</u>- Fresco Burrito Supreme

- <u>Wendy's</u>-Ultimate Chicken Grill (w/o Honey Mustard)

Bonus tip for coffee lovers- A tall, 'skinny' latte has 10-12 grams of protein in it but only about 120 calories. So, go ahead and indulge!

Authors Pick: <u>Chipotle Grill</u>, which is well known for the commitment to organic, local, and sustainable farming practices!

Don't Take My Word For It-Research For Yourself

This is by no means a comprehensive list. I researched well over 200 sources, and have listed just a few of the websites that I found to be reliable and in keeping with consensus. I did not list book titles, as I find most people will use the internet. I read dozens. If you desire to read hardcopies, bookstores and libraries are full of informative writings on the topic of health and nutrition. I did not incorporate material in the book that is not agreed upon by multiple reliable sources, therefore there are no 'diets' listed within these pages. Finally, I did not alphabetize this list of websites. It is assumed that you all know the beginning of websites (www), therefore I omitted this from the listings. Happy reading and researching!

American Heart Association- heart.org

American Diabetes Association-diabetes.org

American Cancer Society-cancer.org

Weight Watchers-weightwatchers.com

rawforbeauty.com

sureyouwanttoeatthat.blogspot.com

simplemom.net

aicr.org

care2.com

everydayroots.com

diseaseproof.com

myfitnesspal.com

organicauthority.com.

prevention.com

thewannabehomesteader.com

blog.naturebox.com

nourishrds.blogspot.com

hubpages.com/hub/foods-that-unclog-arteries

doctoroz.com

health.com

mayoclinic.org

foodnetwork.com

health.usnews.com

abcnews.com

eatingwell.com

healthcentral.com

shape.com

sustainlv.org

medindia.net

seattleorganicrestaurants.net

ask.com

ehow.com

about.com

fda.gov

organicconsumers.org

health.gov

wholefoodsmarket.com

nytimes.com

thebestofrawfood.com

foxnews.com

stonyfield.com

ecoscraps.com

beyondpesticides.org

sustainablelivingassociation.org

sunset.com

facebook.com/growfoodnotlawns

garden.org

organicgardening.com

organiclivingsuperfoods.com

motherearthnews.com

nutrition.gov

homefoodsafety.org

eatright.org

foodallergy.org

organiclivingmag.com

growyourowngroceries.org

theorganicmomma.com

cnn.com

livestrong.com

About the Author

Mel Tavares is an accomplished freelancer who has operated her own company for 15 years and has been contracted as a researcher, technical writer, content writer, and journalist. She has written over 10,000 internet content articles, is a book author, and has written hundreds of newspaper articles for publication. She is an experienced 20 year veteran conference and workshop speaker/teacher.

Mel lives in Middletown, Connecticut with her husband, Joe, and their teenage son. They are all active in their local church. She cherishes time spent with the adult kids and their spouses, as well as all of the grandkids. Her extended family and friends also breathe joy into her, daily.

Her passion is to impart life changing information in oral and written form, to give hope and encouragement to those in search of a more simplistic, healthy and meaningful life. This newest release is another example of her passionate commitment to helping people.

Made in the USA
Charleston, SC
18 September 2014